Mounir Hagui

MEDICAL CERTIFICATE OF FITNESS FOR DIVING IN TUNISIA

Mounir Hagui

MEDICAL CERTIFICATE OF FITNESS FOR DIVING IN TUNISIA

ANALYSISCRITIQUE OF CERTIFICATE-ISSUING PRACTICES

ScienciaScripts

Imprint

Cover image: www.ingimage.com

This book is a translation from the original published under ISBN 978-620-6-72413-1.

Publisher:
Sciencia Scripts
is a trademark of
Dodo Books Indian Ocean Ltd. and OmniScriptum S.R.L publishing group

120 High Road, East Finchley, London, N2 9ED, United Kingdom
Str. Armeneasca 28/1, office 1, Chisinau MD-2012, Republic of Moldova, Europe
Printed at: see last page
ISBN: 978-620-8-15919-1

CONTENTS

Introduction

Scuba diving, long the preserve of professionals, the military and a small number of passionate amateurs, has spread over the last thirty years [1] to become a leisure sport practised all over the world and now open to the whole population, men, women, young people and children. In Tunisia, a country with a coastline some 1300 km long, diving is accessible to a growing number of people. The current population of divers is very heterogeneous in terms of age, physical condition, experience of the underwater environment and interests: leisure, fishing, military activities and large-scale economic projects [2,3].

Despite the fact that scuba diving in Tunisia is governed by regulations that set out the conditions for the practice of diving, in particular with regard to compliance with safety conditions and fitness to practice, a growing number of accidents are noted each year: barotrauma, desaturation accidents, drowning, traumatic accidents, accidents due to gas toxicity [4,5].

Little is known about the epidemiology of scuba diving accidents in Tunisia for several reasons:

1. Absence of a national register of diving accidents which centralises all data relating to the occurrence of diving complications or incidents.

2. Little information is provided on the degree of compliance with the regulations in force and safety conditions in institutions authorised to practice scuba diving (leisure clubs, training centres, companies with professional activities for economic purposes, etc.).

3. A significant number of people continue to dive illegally, fishing at the bottom of the sea and exposing themselves to potentially fatal risks. The Hyperbaric Oxygen Therapy Centre at the Hôpital Militaire Principal d'Instruction in Tunis is witness to the large number of illegal divers admitted to the hyperbaric chamber following a diving accident.

4. The conditions for issuing a medical certificate of fitness or no contraindication to diving in Tunisia are still unclear and subject to numerous disputes, particularly concerning the qualifications of the prescribing doctor and whether divers really respect the obligation to obtain a medical certificate of no contraindication before diving.

The doctor prescribing the fitness to dive has an important role to play in terms of prevention and the protection of human life, through the proper conduct of the interrogation in search of contraindications, through a complete examination and with the help of additional examinations which are essential in order to reach a decision regarding fitness to dive. On the other hand, the absence of a validated model medical certificate that complies with the requirements of the regulations leads to a number of uncertainties when it comes to prescribing medical fitness to dive, whether for leisure or professional purposes.

The aim of our work is to study the practices and conditions for issuing the certificate of aptitude for diving in Tunisia through a survey carried out among divers in order to answer the following two questions:

1. Quantify the proportion of divers with a medical certificate stating that they have no contraindications.

2. To know the qualifications of the doctors who drew up the medical certificates of fitness to dive and the details of the medical examination.

METHODS

1. Type of study :

This is a one-off, prospective, descriptive, multicentre study.

The aim of the study was to evaluate the practices and conditions for issuing diving aptitude certificates in Tunisia.

2. Time and place of the study

The study was carried out during March 2019 and targeted all divers and diving centres available throughout Tunisia.

3. Method, Study design :

We carried out a survey among divers in various diving centres on the procedures for obtaining the certificate of fitness and no contraindications to diving.

The divers surveyed were recruited during meetings of the Tunisian Federation of Underwater and Rescue Activities with its licensed members.

The survey was carried out using a pre-established questionnaire dedicated specifically to the study (Appendix 1).

The questionnaire consisted of 15 questions relating to the epidemiological data of the divers, the conditions, nature and type of diving, frequency of diving, medical check-up and conditions for obtaining a medical certificate, and the occurrence of any complications.

4. Candidates under consideration :

4.1. Inclusion criteria :

All scuba divers were included in the study, regardless of the nature or purpose of their diving.

4.2 Non-inclusion criteria :

No non-inclusion criteria were used.

4.3. Exclusion criteria :

Questionnaires that could not be used, that were incorrectly filled in, or that had been filled in incorrectly, were excluded from the study.
the importance of missing data.

5. Data entry and statistical analysis

The data were analysed using SPSS version 19.0 software and a value of $p<0.05$ was considered statistically significant. Absolute frequencies and relative frequencies were calculated for qualitative variables and means for quantitative variables.

Means and percentages were compared using Student's T and Chi-square parametric tests.

A uni and multivariate analysis using logistic regression and multiple linear regression was used to establish the factors predictive of the occurrence of complications, and in particular the search for a relationship between the quality of the divers' medical follow-up and the risk of complications.

6. Bibliographic research

French and English were used as the research languages.

6.1. Databases used

An exhaustive search for reference texts was carried out on the available databases.

Relevant articles, literature reviews and case studies have been referenced in this work.

The bibliographic search was carried out on the following sites: Sciences Directs, Cochrane net Masson, and the Pubmed search engine.

6.2. Keywords

The keywords used for the bibliographic search were :

Plongée/ Scuba diving

Aptitude/ Aptitude / Medical fitness

Certificat / Certificate

Tunisie / Tunisia

7. Ethical considerations and conflict of interest

We declare that we have no conflict of interest with this study. Authorisation to use data from divers was requested beforehand. Their anonymity was respected. The purpose of the study was explained to them before the questionnaire was administered.

Results

1. Eligibility of patients for the study :

The questionnaire was distributed to divers at 8 dive centres.

After studying the inclusion, non-inclusion and exclusion criteria, 69 questionnaires were selected. The diving centres participating in the study were as follows: Bizerte, Djerba, Haouaria, Hammamet, Mahdia, Monastir, Sousse and Tabarka.

Figure 1 shows the recruitment process for the candidates in the study.

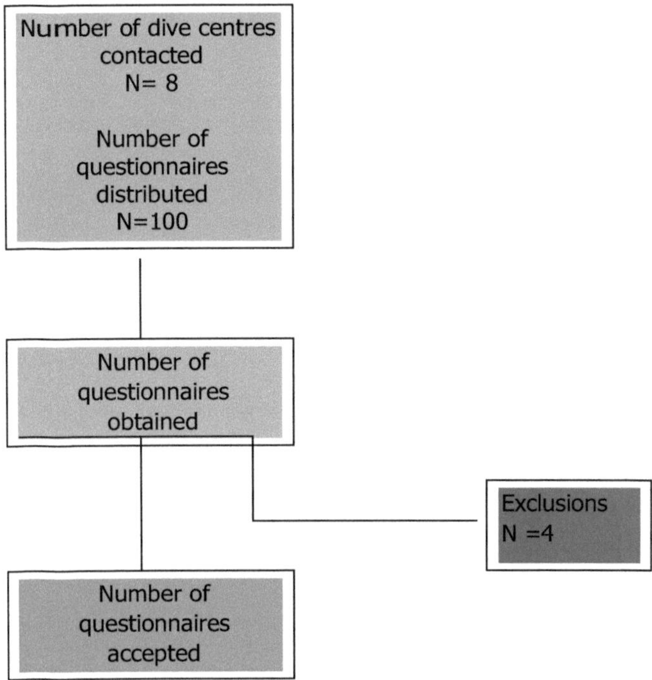

Fig. I: Recruitment of study candidates

2.epidemiological characteristics of the population

2.1. Age

The average age of the study population was 41.95 [17-62] years, with more than half of the divers aged over 40 (58%), as shown in Figure 2.

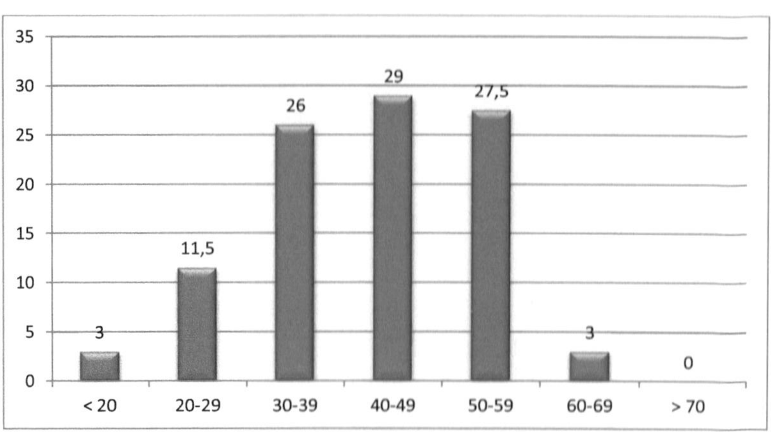

Fig. II: Distribution of divers according to age.

2.2 Gender

Of the 69 divers included in our study, only one woman took part in the survey, corresponding to a female participation rate of 1.45%.

2.3 Type of dive

In our study, three types of diving activities were identified:

- Sport diving
- Recreational diving (amateur divers)
- Professional diving

Sport diving was the most frequently practised activity in our study (45%)

In less than 2% of cases, the diver was involved in two types of activity

Table 1 summarises the distribution of divers by type of activity.

Table 1: Distribution of divers by type of activity.

Type of diver	N=	%
Professional diving	21	30,5%
Leisure activity (Amateur)	16	23 %
Sports activity	31	45%
Professional + sports	1	1,5%
Total	69	100 %

2.4. Nature of professional diving

Of the 22 professional divers included in our study, half were coral divers or coral diver instructors (50%),

The breakdown of professional divers according to the nature of their activity is shown in Table 2.

Table 2: Breakdown of professional divers according to the nature of their activity

Type of profession	N=	%
Corailleur	9	41
Diving instructor	8	36,5
Trainer of corailleurs	2	9
Maritime works, topography, geomatics	3	13,5
Total	22	100 %

2.5. Diving site

In our study, two thirds (65%) of diving activities were located in the northern region of Tunisia, with the three most frequently used sites for diving being Tabarka, Hammamet and El Haouaria. The Tunis region was not included in our data, as the regional diving club did not participate in the survey. In 16% of cases, the divers' activity was multi-site in different regions of Tunisia. Table 3 details the distribution of regions where diving activities were carried out.

Table 3: Breakdown of diving activities by region

Region	Dive Site	Workforce	%	% by region
North-East region	Bizerte	7	11	33
	Hammamet - Haouaria	15	22	
North-West Region	Tabarka	22	32	32
Centre-East Region	Monastir	3	4	12
	Mahdia	4	5	
	Sousse	2	3	
South-East region	Zarzis - Djerba	5	7	7
Multi-site	Several regions	11	16	16
	Total	69	100	100

2.6. Seniority in diving

The length of time people had been diving varied greatly. In 38.5% of cases, divers had been diving for less than 15 years. In 45.5% of cases, the divers had been diving for more than 25 years.

The average length of service was 20.27 [2-40] years.

Figure 3 shows the distribution of divers according to how long they have been diving.

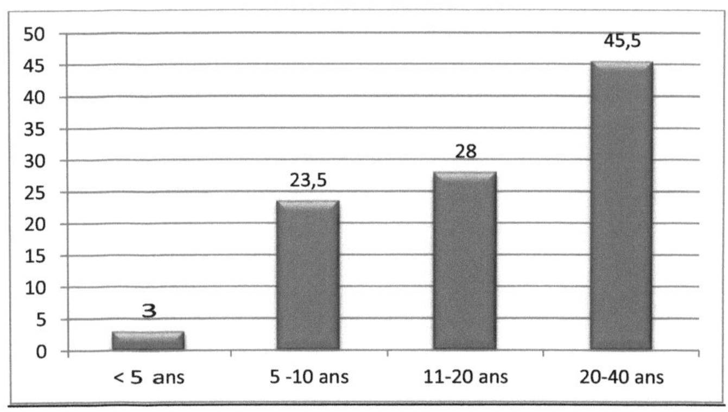

Fig. III: Distribution of divers according to how long they have been diving

2.7. Dive frequency

Dive frequency is defined as the number of dives made in number of days per year [6].

In our study, we found several groups of divers, depending on how often they dive:

1. Divers who dive less than 10 times a year (N= 23), i.e. a rate of 34%.

2. Divers with a diving frequency of less than 3 months (N=22), i.e. a rate of 32%.

3. Diving activity varying between 3 and 6 months a year: 8%.

4. Divers who dive a lot for more than 6 months a year with a frequency of once a day every day of the week to several times a day (N= 24), i.e. a rate of 26%.

Figure IV shows the distribution of divers according to frequency of activity.

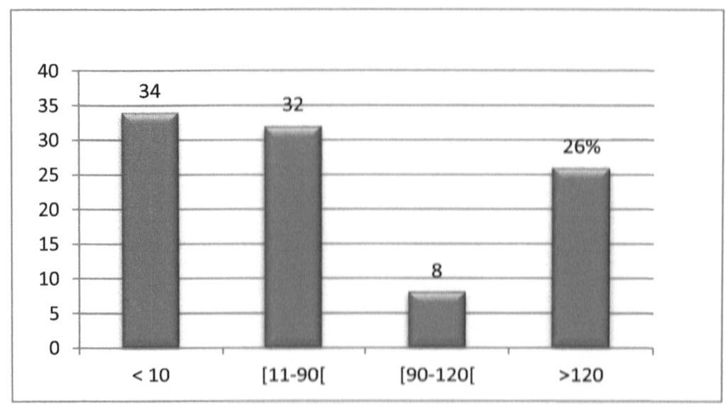

Fig.IV : Distribution of divers according to frequency of activity

3. Medical examination and medical certificate of fitness to dive

3.1. Obtaining a medical certificate of fitness to dive

In our study, 62 of the 69 divers questioned obtained a certificate of no contraindication to diving, a rate of 91%.

In 9% of cases, i.e. 7 divers did not have a medical check-up before diving, these were 4 professional divers, 4 amateur divers and two sport divers. Figure 5 shows the distribution of divers according to medical clearance for diving.

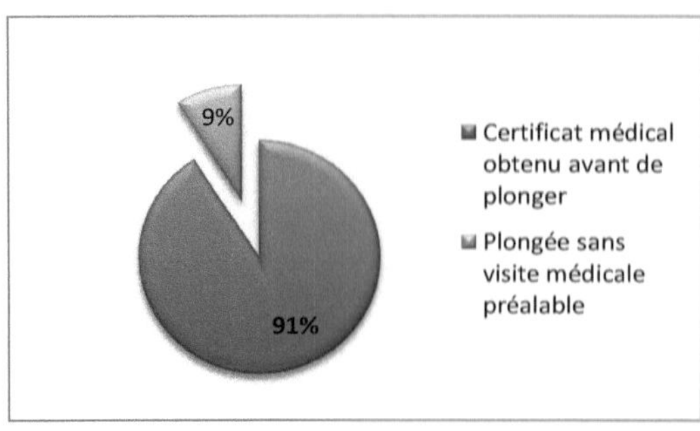

Fig. V: Distribution of divers according to medical diving authorisation.

3.2. Age of first medical certificate of fitness to dive

In our study, only 8% of divers had a diving certificate that was less than 5 years old. In more than half the cases, the certificate was more than 20 years old.

Table 4 shows the distribution of divers according to the age of their first medical certificate of fitness to dive.

Table 4: Age of first medical certificate

Age of first medical certificate (years)	N=	%
0- 5	5	8
6-10	12	19
11-20	19	31
> 20	26	42
Total	**62**	**100**

3.3. Qualification of the doctor issuing the medical certificate of fitness to dive

In our study, more than two thirds of the divers used a general practitioner to obtain a medical certificate stating that they were fit or not contraindicated to dive (71%).

Only 13 divers (21%) used the services of a doctor qualified in underwater and hyperbaric medicine.

Table 5 shows the distribution of doctors issuing diving certificates according to medical speciality.

Table 5: Medical competence of the doctor issuing the diving certificate.

Doctor's speciality	Workforce	Percentage
General practitioner	44	71%

Doctor with expertise in underwater and hyperbaric medicine	13	21%
ENT specialist	3	5%
Doctor with expertise in sports medicine	2	3%
Total	62	100%

3.4. Renewal rate for initial medical certificate

In our study, only 19 divers (30%) stated that they had renewed their medical certificate of no contraindication to diving at least once. In the vast majority of cases (70%), the initial certificate had not been renewed.

Table 6 shows the distribution of divers according to the renewal of their diving certificate.

Table 6: Distribution of divers according to renewal of diving certificate.

Renewal of medical certificate of no contraindication to diving	Workforce	Percentage
No	43	70%
Yes	19	30%
Total	62	100 %

3.5. Qualification of the doctor issuing the renewal of the medical certificate of fitness to dive

In our study, only 19 divers (28%) had their medical certificate renewed.

In 58% of cases, the renewal was carried out by a GP.

Table 7: Competence of the doctor issuing the renewal of the medical certificate of fitness to dive

The doctor's competence	Workforce	Percentage
General practitioner	11	58%
Sports doctor	3	16%
General practitioner with expertise in underwater medicine	2	10%
Specialist	3	16%
Total	19	100%

3.6. The prescribing doctor according to sector of activity

In our study, only one diver in four used a public health doctor to obtain a medical certificate of no contraindication to diving, while 75% of divers obtained their medical certificate from a doctor practising in the private sector.

Table 8 shows the distribution of prescribing doctors by sector of activity.

Table 8: Breakdown of prescribing doctors by sector of activity.

Physician's sector of activity	Workforce	Percentage
Free practice doctor	46	75 %
Public Sector Doctor	16	25 %
Total	62	100 %

3.7. Frequency of renewal of the medical certificate of non-contraindication to diving

The medical certificate of fitness was renewed by only 19 of the 62 divers who obtained an initial diving certificate, a rate of 30.5%.

In 10 cases, only one renewal was carried out, representing a rate of

This visit was only made once during the entire period of diving activity for ten people, i.e. 14.71% of the series.

Table 9: Frequency of renewal of the medical certificate of non-contraindication to diving

Frequency of medical check-ups	Workforce	%
Only once	10	53%
Once a year	1	5%
Once / 2 years	3	16%
Once/5 years	5	26%
Total	19	100%

4. The medical examination for non-contraindication to diving

4.1. Medical check-up

The clinical examination consisted of an interview and a search for pathological history in 100% of cases (n=69).

A medical examination of the diver was carried out in only 52% of cases.

A specialist ENT examination was requested in 30.5% of cases only. Audiometry and impedancemetry were requested in 9.2% and 7.6% of cases respectively.

4.2. Additional examinations

In 80% of cases (n=49), no further examination was requested by the doctor issuing the diving certificate.

Table 10 gives details of the percentage of para-clinical examinations requested during medical fitness tests.

Table 10: Type of additional examination carried out during the medical check-up

	Type of examination	**N=**	**%**
1.	Biological blood tests	8	13
2.	X-ray of the lung	13	21
3.	Osteoarticular radiological assessment	9	14,5
4.	EFR	6	9,5
5.	ECG	6	9,5
6.	Exercise test	8	13
7.	EEG	5	8
8.	Hyperbaric chamber test	8	13

5. Prevalence of diving accidents

The prevalence of diving accidents in our study was 19%. In our series, 56 divers, or 81% of cases, stated that they had never had a diving accident.

Table 11: Breakdown of diving accidents by type of accident

Nature of the diving accident	**N=**	**%**
Atrial barotrauma	2	15,5
Desaturation accident	4	31
Discomfort	2	15,5
Alternating episodes of vertigo	5	38

	Total	13	100%

5.1. Characteristics of divers involved in diving accidents.

The average age of divers involved in diving accidents was 52.61 [42-62] years. All were men.

The average time spent scuba diving was 31.53 years.

Among the 13 divers who suffered a diving accident, we counted 8 professionals and 5 sportsmen and women. The frequency of diving was greater than 6 months per year for 12 divers, a rate of 92%. 52% of the divers were core divers.

All the divers had an initial medical certificate of fitness to dive. The certificate was dated on average 28 [15-32] years ago. Only 39% of the divers had renewed their certificate at least once during the entire period of diving. In 3 out of 4 cases, the certificate was issued by a general practitioner.

The number of divers who benefited from hyperbaric chamber sessions was 7, a rate of 54%.

6. Predictors of complications: correlation study

6.1. Univariate study

we carried out a univariate study to determine the variables that could influence the occurrence of diving accidents.

The variables included were :

1. Age
2. Age of dive
3. Dive frequency
4. medical certificate of fitness yes/no
5. Certificate renewal yes/no
6. Type of activity (sporting, professional, amateur)
7. Medical certificate without clinical examination
8. Medical certificate + clinical examination only
9. Medical certificate with additional examinations
10. Patients' medical history

In univariate analysis, 3 variables were significantly correlated with the occurrence of complications. These were professional diving, more than 20 years of diving and more than 4 months of diving per year.

Variable	***OR***	***P Value***
1. Professional diving	1,87 [1,53-4]	<0,05
2. Age of diving > 20 years	2,87 [2,00-3,14]	<0,05
3. Frequency of diving > 120d/year	1,43 [1,21-1,89]	<0,02

6.2. Multi-variate study

The multivariate study showed that only the frequency of diving > 120 times/year was significantly correlated with the occurrence of complications (OR: 2.8 [1.32- 6.00]).

No correlation was found with the divers' medical conditions or with whether or not they had a certificate authorising them to dive.

Discussion

Our study focused on the conditions for issuing medical certificates of fitness and non-disqualification for diving and the medical monitoring of divers in Tunisia.

In our series, diving was mainly for sport (45%), with professional diving accounting for only 30.5% of cases. Recreational diving accounted for 23% of diving activities.

Diving was the preserve of men, with a rate of 98.5%.

In 85% of cases, the divers were aged over 30.

Half of the professional divers surveyed were coral divers or coral diver instructors (50%). The average length of time they had been diving was 20, 27 [2-40] years.

The prevalence of complications in our series was 19%, and included atrial barotrauma, decompression accidents with neurological damage, dyspnoea and malaise.

85.5% of divers had obtained a certificate of fitness to dive at least once. 14.5% of divers had never obtained a certificate of fitness to dive or of no contraindication to diving. In 52% of cases, the initial certificate of fitness to dive was more than 20 years old and in 72% of cases, no re-assessment of fitness had been carried out since the first certificate.

In 78% of cases, the certificate of fitness to dive was issued by a general practitioner who was not qualified in underwater and hyperbaric medicine.

In 75% of cases, the certificate was issued by an independent doctor.

The medical assessment of the diver during the fitness visit consisted essentially of a brief clinical examination, and an ENT examination was requested in 1/3 of cases. Radiological, biological and functional tests were requested in less than 15% of cases.

The uni and multivariate studies carried out in parallel with our work showed no correlation between medical follow-up and the risk of complications.

We can thus draw up a profile of the Tunisian diver; this is a man aged over 40 with over 20 years' experience, a professional or sportsman who has only once obtained a medical certificate of fitness during a medical interview with a general practitioner with no expertise in underwater and hyperbaric medicine, consisting of a summary clinical examination and sometimes an additional ENT examination.

1. Highlights of the study

Our study is the first to be carried out in Tunisia with the aim of evaluating medical practices in the care of divers and the conditions under which medical certificates are issued. This is a topical issue for the authorities involved in scuba diving in Tunisia.

2. weaknesses of the study

Although our study addressed a relevant subject, certain shortcomings should be noted.

Our study included a limited number of divers, which is not representative of the population of divers in Tunisia. The Fédération Tunisienne des Activités Subaquatiques alone has 400 members [4]. The questionnaire relating to our study was distributed to several diving clubs, but the number of divers who responded was very limited (N=69). No diver from the Greater Tunis region responded to our study.

We noted that there was a selection bias, as the questionnaire only targeted the most accessible divers; due to a problem of distance, the distribution of the questionnaire was not unequivocal, as some divers were contacted at FAST meetings in different regions, while others were contacted by email.

It would have been wiser to interview the divers directly to explain some of the information they had misunderstood. We found that some divers did not master all the aspects of diving, the procedures to follow and, above all, the different types of possible complications.

3. Epidemiological data on divers

In our study, the average age of the divers interviewed was 42 [17-62] years, with divers aged over 50 representing 30% of the population studied. This trend towards an ageing population of divers is partly due to the absence of an upper age limit for diving, especially for professional divers [7]. For non-professionals, diving is a highly sought-after sport after retirement, which explains why a large number of people take up this activity at a very advanced age [7].

The phenomenon of an ageing population of divers has also been observed in other studies [2,6,8]. In the series by Plancoulaine et al [8], which included 519 divers, the average age was 47 [40-59] years. However, most studies agree that the general population of divers worldwide remains relatively young [6, 7, 8] (Table 11).

Table 11: Average age of divers by series worldwide

Study	Country	N=	Average age (years)
Bonnans et al [7]	France (2001)	289	42
Plancoulaine et al[8].	France (2017)	310	47
Clara et al [6]	Reunion Island (2008)	519	36,5
Faralli et al [2]	Italy (2003)	60	32
Our study	Tunisia	69	42

In terms of gender, our series included only one woman (rate < 1.5%); diving in Tunisia remains the preserve of men, whatever the nature of the activities undertaken at sea [4]. In Tunisia, we do not have exact data on the diver population. The websites of the Tunisian Federation of Subaquatic and Rescue Activities (FAST) and the Tunisian Federation of Nautical Tourism Activities (FTANT) do not provide any information on divers.

In France (2017 data) [6,8], 30% of the certifications of the French federation of underwater activities were awarded to women, who represent 27% of the diving population [6].

4. Characteristics of diving in Tunisia

In our study, half of the professional divers were coral divers (50%), despite the fact that coral fishing is a seasonal activity in Tunisia (opening of the season), the questionnaire revealed that these coral divers dived throughout the year, travelling outside the Tunisian borders, mainly to Algeria during the opening of the season elsewhere.

A detailed analysis of the epidemiology of diving in Tunisia cannot be made in the absence of published data, and we noted a complete absence of data relating to divers in Tunisia during our bibliographic search carried out as part of our study. The data from our series (n= 69) cannot be representative of the population of divers in Tunisia. We estimate that our series represents less than 10% of the total number of divers.

In our series, the average length of diving experience in Tunisia was 20.27 years, with extremes ranging from 2 to 40 years. These were mainly professional and sports divers, 68% of whom had been diving for more than 3 months.

The results of our study suggest that diving in Tunisia is the preserve of professionals and high-level sportsmen and women; few young people in Tunisia are interested in diving as a sporting or leisure activity. We cannot confirm these findings in the absence of a wider database and reliable statistics. Is this a Tunisian exception? Worldwide, diving is a rapidly expanding activity among young people, all activities included [1,2 ,4,5,6 ,8,9].

5. Diving accidents and complications

The prevalence of diving accidents in our series was 19%. The accidents were auricular barotrauma, desaturation accidents with neurological deficit, malaise and transient episodes of vertigo. The diving accidents occurred in professional divers aged over 50, with more than 30 years' experience and a diving frequency of more than 6 months per year. They were mainly coral divers. All the divers had an initial medical certificate of fitness to dive issued by a general practitioner that was more than 20 years old in more than two-thirds of cases, with a renewal rate of 39%. We believe that this figure is an underestimate of the exact number of diving accidents in our series, as some divers avoided reporting their complications, while others were unaware that certain pathologies were indeed secondary complications of diving.

The prevalence of diving accidents was 8.1% in the Clara et al study [6] and 19.3% in the Plancoulaine study.

6. Procedure for obtaining a medical certificate

In our study, 91% of the divers had a first medical certificate of fitness to dive at the very beginning of their Level 1 training or during a first dive. In 9% of cases, the diver had never obtained medical clearance to dive, despite being a licensed diver. In 80% of cases, the medical certificate was more than 10 years old. In our series, we identified 4 professional coral divers in the informal sector (6% of divers) who were not affiliated to a health insurance fund. Of the 3 groups of divers identified (professionals, sports divers and amateurs), it was the sports divers who benefited most from close medical monitoring (100% initial certificate of fitness, 87% renewal).

In a study carried out on Reunion Island [6], Clara et al. reported that in 40% of cases, the renewal of the medical certificate of fitness was not up to date because the clubs and employing organisations did not require it in a third of cases, and in 2 thirds of cases, the diver himself considered himself to be in good health or the doctor refused to issue it because of a contraindication.

Diving in Tunisia remains a poorly organised sector despite the existence of laws governing the practice of scuba diving activities, and few arguments were put forward by divers when the questionnaire was carried out. Informally, several divers did not consider it necessary to undergo a medical examination for fear of being banned from diving.

7. Regulations in Tunisia

In Tunisia, diving is essentially governed by decrees relating to scuba diving in addition to the labour code for professional divers. This activity is supervised by the Ministry of Youth and Sport, as well as the Ministry of Social Affairs and the Ministry of Agriculture for professional divers [10,11,12,13,14,15].

7.1. Professional diving

It is governed by the Labour Code and two ministerial decrees, decree no. 2008-2568 of 7 July 2008 and decree no. 68-83 of 23/3/1968 on work requiring special medical supervision, as well as the laws on compensation for damage resulting from accidents at work and occupational diseases for the private sector, which stipulate [11,12,13,15,16]:

- Divers must have a medical logbook.

- The medical check-up is an annual event, and is stepped up if necessary.

- In the event of a diving accident, a declaration must be made to the occupational health inspector.

- The certificate of fitness and of no contraindication to diving, or of temporary or permanent cessation of diving, is issued by an occupational physician on the advice of a physician with competence in diving medicine [11].

Article 13 of the aforementioned decree no. 2008-2568 stipulates that: "In order to practice diving professionally as a physiologically demanding activity, especially from a cardiovascular, pulmonary, otorhinolaryngological and neurological point of view, the following general conditions of medical fitness must be met:

- the absence of any cardiovascular or pulmonary disease,
- the absence of any condition that may affect the ability to equalise pressure in the lungs, middle ear and sinuses,
- the absence of any disease that could lead to sudden loss of consciousness.

The decrees specify that a medical examination of fitness to dive professionally is compulsory periodically and after any diving accident or intercurrent illness. All professional divers must undergo special medical monitoring.

It should be noted that in Tunisia, the procedures for carrying out the aforementioned medical examinations, the list of additional examinations, the medical tests and the criteria for fitness to dive professionally are laid down by joint order of the Minister for Public Health and the Minister for Occupational Medicine and Safety.

7.2. Recreational diving

Decree no. 2008-2568 of 7 July 2008 stipulates [11]:

- Divers must have a medical logbook.

- No medical certificate is required for dives to a depth of less than 2 metres.

- A medical certificate of fitness is required for all four performance levels

- In the event of an accident, the accident is reported to the health inspector.

- the medical check-up is periodic and after every diving accident

- No qualification is required (not specified) for the prescribing doctor.

8. The prescribing doctor

In Tunisia, competence in diving medicine is obtained by obtaining a certificate of complementary studies in underwater and hyperbaric medicine from the Tunis Faculty of Medicine and registering with the National Medical Council (CNOM), which recognises the holder of the certificate as competent in diving medicine.

The doctor holding the certificate of complementary studies in sports medicine is also authorised to issue the certificate of fitness to dive, despite the fact that the certificate does not include any training in diving medicine.

The doctor specialising in occupational medicine is authorised to treat divers as part of the monitoring of professional workers in an underwater environment. The decree stipulates the need to refer to a doctor qualified in underwater medicine if necessary [11].

Decree no. 2008-2568 of 7 July 2008 and decree no. 68-83 of 23/3/1968 relating to work requiring special medical supervision stipulate that fitness to dive in a professional capacity must be declared by the occupational physician following the opinion of a physician with recognised competence in diving medicine [11,15].

In our study, 69% of divers consulted a general practitioner. In less than 10% of cases, a doctor with expertise in diving medicine was consulted.

In the Clara et al. study, the general practitioner was used in only 3% of cases. In 45.5% of cases, it was the doctor specialising in diving medicine, and in 42% of cases, the doctor prescribing the fitness test was the attending physician [6].

In his study, Faralli reported that the certificate of fitness to dive was issued by a doctor specialising in diving medicine in 100% of cases [2].

In France, Thomas et al. found that the federal doctor was called in 39% of cases [8].

In Morocco [17], a qualification in diving medicine is not required to issue a certificate of fitness to dive, the joint decree of 1962, (n°212-61 of 25 July 1962 relating to the conditions of physical fitness to be met for the practice of swimming or underwater fishing) authorises all Moroccan doctors to issue the medical certificate to divers, with **recommendations from the Minister of Public** Health **relating to the medical examination of persons wishing to practice underwater fishing, which state that this examination** may, if the doctor deems it necessary for the safety of the subject, be completed by an examination carried out by a specialist doctor.

During the course of our study we noted a series of constraints reported by divers relating to recourse to a specialist diving doctor:

- lack of information from the divers surveyed and lack of follow-up by employers (diving clubs, hoteliers and other company managers)

- the geographical distribution and demography of doctors specialising in diving medicine is unknown, poorly catalogued and badly distributed.

We report that a project by the FTASS national medical and prevention commission is currently being drawn up to establish a list of doctors qualified in diving medicine and to distribute this list to clubs and organisations working in the field of scuba diving.

9. Medical examination for fitness to dive

In our series, we noted a disparity in the attitudes of the doctors concerning the content of the clinical examination and the request for complementary examinations, which remains below the standards recommended for the care of divers in Tunisia. In 48% of cases, the medical examination consisted simply of an interview about the patient's state of health and previous history, and a brief clinical examination was carried out in only 52% of cases. In only 30% of cases was a specialist ENT examination requested. A complementary examination was prescribed in only 15% of cases.

We also found that :

- there is no distinction between the initial medical check-up and the annual assessment.

- no consideration is given to the diver's level of technical skill, the nature of his activity or his individual characteristics, particularly as regards age.

When questioned, some divers reported that they preferred to go to the general practitioner of their choice simply to obtain the certificate without undergoing a medical examination. We cannot extrapolate or generalise from this observation due to the lack of objective data.

In Tunisia, the Ministry of Agriculture provides training in the form of the Brevet de Technicien Professionnel Plongeur subaquatique (professional diploma in underwater diving) awarded by the Agence de la Vulgarisation et de la Formation Agricole (agricultural extension and training agency), which states on its website that the conditions for enrolment in the diploma are limited to producing a medical certificate in accordance with a model provided by the establishment [18], justifying the physical aptitudes required to practise the speciality in question and passing a test of behaviour at sea during an appropriate period of pre-selection training, the terms of which are set by the class council. No mention is made of the qualifications of the prescribing doctor, nor of the need to consult an occupational physician, even though this is a professional activity and a recruitment examination.

In France, to practice diving, the FFESSM requires the production of a medical certificate of fitness and no contraindications to diving (CACI) less than one year old according to the decree of 24 July 2017 on disciplines with special constraints. It is mentioned in its first paragraph, common to all disciplines, that the medical examination must be carried out by a competent doctor (who has the knowledge, experience and means to do so, in accordance with Article 70 of the Code of Ethics) and in accordance with good practice recommendations, in particular those of the French Society of Exercise and Sport Medicine (SFMES). The initial medical examination for fitness includes an interview, a clinical examination and a cardiovascular assessment based on a health questionnaire and a clinical and complementary examination form[19].

The FTASS and the FFESSM state that it is the doctor's responsibility to assess the need to carry out the examinations he or she deems necessary.
[4,19,20] although the medical decision on fitness is a matter of medical responsibility [30].
Across the world, the treatment of divers for fitness to dive is nuanced, and the signed self-questionnaire on medical history is very useful [21,22, 24,25,26,27,31] . In France, the 2016 and 2018 recommendations of the French Society of Sub-aquatic and Hyperbaric Medicine and Physiology and the French Society of Occupational Medicine for the occupational health management of workers involved in hyperbaric conditions recommend carrying out a medical examination from the age of 40 [21-23] :

- An annual medical check-up with functional respiratory exploration (recording of flow-volume curves) and a resting electrocardiogram

- A stress test is indicated in subjects at risk;

- Additional tests may be prescribed on request to investigate the long-term effects of hyperbaric exposure [22].

Plancoulaine [8], in his study of 519 divers and the risk of complications, suggested adapting the request for complementary examinations according to the diver's age:

- An ECG, at the time of the initial aptitude test, then every 3 years between 12 and 20 years of practice, and every 5 years after 20 years of practice.

- A chest X-ray is taken at the initial examination, and is then taken if necessary.

- Visual acuity tests are carried out annually for level 3 and 4 professional divers.

- Biological tests containing a blood count and platelet count, a lipid profile, fasting blood sugar levels, a urine dipstick and a kidney function test should be carried out regularly.

- A stress test is recommended after the age of 35 if you resume diving. After the age of 59, a stress test should be carried out if there are cardiovascular risk factors, and repeated every 5 years.

- Audio-tympanometry should be carried out regularly for divers under the age of 14 and for people over the age of 59.

These practices are generally accepted and are found in the United Kingdom [28] as well as in other international bodies such as the PADI International Association of Diving Instructors [28- 32,33].

10. Recommendations

Following this critical analysis of the conditions under which the medical certificate of fitness to dive is issued, we propose to put forward recommendations from our point of view with a view to improving the medical care of divers in Tunisia.

- Draw up a declaration of honour form concerning the diver's medical history, using a self-questionnaire to retrace the diver's medical history, in order to encourage the diver to sign and commit to protecting his or her health. This form will be presented at the beginning of the medical check-up.

- To raise awareness among divers and all professionals working in the underwater environment of the importance of the medical certificate of fitness and the risks incurred if regular medical check-ups are not carried out as required by law.

- To raise awareness among those involved in diving (sports and leisure clubs, employers) of the importance of keeping a diver's logbook and complying with the requirements contained therein.

- Establish a protocol for the medical care of senior divers adapted to the anatomical and physiological particularities of the elderly subject.

- Establish stricter medical surveillance requirements for diving professionals, depending on the diver's technical skills, the frequency of diving and the nature of the underwater activities.

- Draw up a list of doctors authorised to provide diving fitness certificates who have obtained competence in underwater medicine, distribute this list to professionals and all organisations working in the underwater field and insist that only competence in underwater medicine authorises the prescription of a medical certificate of fitness to dive.

- Continuing medical training for general practitioners in diving medicine and the requirements of the medical certificate of aptitude (these doctors are the first point of contact for divers) and creating a network of prescribing doctors attached to the Tunisian federation.

- Encourage the public bodies organising the sector to publish the implementing decrees relating to the medical certificate and aptitude set out in decree no. 2008-2568 of 7 July 2008 as soon as possible. This measure would make a major contribution to the organisation of diving activities.
- To agree on the need to draw up different standardised models of medical certificates that take into account the specific characteristics of the different categories of divers, depending on the nature of the authorised activities.

- We therefore propose a 3-stage model for the medical examination:

1. The purpose of this Medical Questionnaire is to determine whether it is necessary to consult a doctor before taking part in diving training, particularly for recreational purposes. The diver undertakes to declare that the information provided on his/her medical history is accurate.

2. A complete and detailed clinical examination backed up by targeted complementary examinations depending on the type of visit (initial or annual), the diver's technical skills and individual characteristics.

3. a time for prevention At the end of the consultation, the doctor must organise a session aimed at prevention, providing information and raising awareness of the importance of the medical examination for fitness to dive and no contraindication to diving, regular medical monitoring and compliance with the recommendations and requirements of the regulations, and must provide the diver with hygienic and dietary advice to prevent metabolic diseases and other health risks.

Conclusions

The practice of subaquatic and hyperbaric activities is expanding rapidly throughout the world, whatever the nature of the activities undertaken in the underwater environment. Diving can cause the decompensation of pre-existing pathologies, as well as specific immediate or long-term accidents. The medical monitoring of divers is based on a preventive approach based on the strict application of specific medical surveillance.

The decision on medical fitness to dive is a medical responsibility and must be based on scientifically proven and regulatory arguments.

The aim of our work was to analyse the conditions for issuing the medical certificate of fitness to dive in Tunisia and to specify the practical procedures for carrying out this surveillance. We also proposed a series of recommendations in the light of our findings, with the aim of better defining the problem of the medical follow-up of divers in Tunisia.

We carried out a descriptive observational study using a self-questionnaire survey of 69 divers, focusing on their medical follow-up and the procedures for obtaining a medical certificate of fitness to dive.

In our study, the average age of divers in all categories was 42 [17-62] years, with a clear predominance of males; only one woman was recorded in our series. We observed an ageing population of divers in Tunisia, a fact that is not isolated; several studies have reported the same finding.

In terms of length of diving experience, the average was 21 years, with only 3% of divers having less than 5 years' experience.

Sport diving was predominant in our series (48%), with professional divers accounting for a third of the series, 50% of whom were coral divers.

The rate of complications inherent in scuba diving was 19% (13 cases), in the form of auricular barotrauma, desaturation accidents, alternating episodes of vertigo and recurrent malaise.

The study of the frequency of diving enabled us to distinguish essentially 3 groups of divers, a first category of divers whose frequency of diving was less than 10 dives per year (34%), a second category with a frequency of 3 to 6 months of activity per year (33%) and in 33% of cases, the frequency of diving was greater than 6 months per year.

The initial medical certificate of fitness to dive was obtained by 85.5% of divers. In 14.5% of cases, the diver had never obtained a medical certificate authorising him or her to dive.

The initial medical certificate was less than 5 years old in only 8% of cases. In 50% of cases, the initial certificate of fitness to dive was more than 20 years old.

The rate of renewal of the medical certificate of fitness was 30%.

In 71% of cases, the certificate was issued by a general practitioner who was not qualified in underwater and hyperbaric medicine. The certificate was prescribed in the private sector in 75% of cases.

The medical examination for fitness to dive consisted of a medical history in 48% of cases, and a complementary clinical examination was carried out in 52% of cases. A specialist ENT opinion was requested in only 30% of cases. Additional tests were requested in only 15% of cases.

No correlation was found in our univariate and multivariate study between the risk of complications and the diver's medical conditions or whether or not the diver had a certificate authorising diving.

Following our critical analysis of the conditions under which the medical certificate of fitness to dive is issued in Tunisia, we have made a number of recommendations designed to provide our point of view on the issue of the medical certificate of fitness to dive, with a view to improving the medical care of divers in Tunisia.

References

1. Pugin D, Berney JY. Scuba diving and hyperbaric medicine. Rev Med Suisse 2009; 5: 1610-4. Available online at https://www.revmed.ch/RMS/2009/RMS-213/Plongee-sous-marine-et-medecine-hyperbare

2. Farralli F, Panico S, Renzoni S, Cardoni F, Pultrone V et al. Analysis of scuba diving accidents in a hyperbaric treatment centre. An Italian study. Documents pour le médecin du travail. 2ème trimestre 2003; n° 94: 171-81

3. Abouda M. Freediving accidents and means of prevention in Tunisia [Thesis]. Master de Médecine de plongée et hyperbare : Tunis;2012 .28 pages.

4. Fédération Tunisienne des Activités Subaquatiques et de Sauvetage [online : 2006] [2 screens] available at http://www.fast.org.tn/histofast.asp

5. Rebai M H. Les Accidents De Plongée Sous- Marine : Etude De 18 Cas [Mémoire]. CEC en Médecine Subaquatique et Hyperbare : Tunis;2013 .54 pages.

6. Galaup C. Diving and health: an epidemiological study of 519 divers on Reunion Island [Thesis]. Medical sciences: Bordeaux; 2017. N°190. 92 pages. Available at URL https://dumas.ccsd.cnrs.fr/dumas-01658768/document

7. Szalay Bonnans E. Diving among seniors. Association réunionnaise de médecine subaquatique et hyperbare .Table Ronde de Médecine de Plongée de l'Océan Indien. 10 and 11 October 2001. Mauritius. Available at www.aresub.org

8. PlancoulaineT.Enquête de pratique autour du certificat de non contreindication à la pratique de la plongée sous-marine dans la grande métropole lilloise [thèse] . Lille 2 ; 2017 .97 pages .Available at URL http://pepite.univ-lille2.fr/notice/view/UDSL2-workflow-9425

9. Ben Dhia I E. Causes médicales d'inaptitude définitive à la plongée professionnelle [Mémoire]. Mastère Spécialisé En Médecine Subaquatique Et Hyperbare : Tunis;2005 .44 pages.

10. Republic of Tunisia. Law 2005-89 of 3 October 2005 on the organisation of diving activities, Official Gazette of the Republic of Tunisia No. 79 of 4 October 2005, p. 25872.

11. Republic of Tunisia. Decree No. 2008-2568 of 7 July 2008 laying down the conditions of medical and technical fitness and the terms and conditions of diving activities. Journal officiel de la république Tunisienne N° 57 du 15 juillet 2008 p 2114

12. République Tunisienne .loi 66-27 du 30 avril 1996 modifiée par la loi n° 96-62 du 15 juillet 1996 et la loi 2006-18 du 2 mai 2006, concernant le Code du Travail Tunisien. Journal officiel de la république Tunisienne n°20 des 3 et 6 mai 1966 p 716

13. Republic of Tunisia. Decree No. 2000-1985 of 12 September 2000, on the organisation and operation of occupational medicine services. Journal officiel de la république Tunisienne n° 076 du 22/09/2000

14. République Tunisienne .Décret fixant les prérogatives, la composition et les règles de fonctionnement de la commission nationale de plongée. Official Journal of the Republic of Tunisia n° 2006-1017 of 13 April 2006

15. République Tunisienne .Décret n° 68-83 du 23 mars 1968 fixant la nature des travaux nécessitant une surveillance médicale spéciale décrété par le secrétaire d'état à la jeunesse , aux sports et aux affaires sociales .Journal officiel de la république Tunisienne du 23 mars 1968

16. République Tunisienne .loi N°94-28 du 21 février 1994 Portant régime de réparation des préjudices résultant des accidents de travail et des maladies professionnelles. Journal officiel de la république Tunisienne No. 15 of 22 February 1994, pages 308-318

17. Kingdom of Morocco. Joint order of the Minister of Commerce, Industry, Mines, Handicrafts and the Merchant Navy and the Minister of Public Health. Bulletin Officiel

Marocain n° 2604 du 21 septembre 1962 n° 212-61 du 25 juillet 1962 relatif aux conditions d'aptitude Physique à remplir pour la pratique de la pêche à la nage ou pêche Sous-marine.

18. Agricultural extension and training agency. Formation initiale pêche Brevet de technicien professionnel plongeur subaquatique [On line].Ministère de l'Agriculture [Mai 2019/ mis à jour 2008] ; [1 écran]. Available from URL: http://www.avfa.agrinet.tn/fr/descriptionform2.php?code=17

19. Fédération Française d'Etudes et de Sports Sous Marins. Certificat médical d'absence de contre-indication à la pratique des activités subaquatiques [cited 10/4/ 2019]; available from URL http://medical.ffessm.fr/wp-content/uploads/CMPN-mod%C3%A8le-de-certificat-m%C3%A9dical-V9.pdf

20. French Federation of Underwater Studies and Sports FFESSM. Commissions Médicale et de Prévention. Règlement Médical /chapitre III - surveillance médicale des licenciés .Paris : FFESSM février ; 2018 14 pages online at http://medical.ffessm.fr

21. Société de médecine et de physiologie subaquatiques et hyperbares de langue française (MEDSUBHYP) Société française de médecine du travail (SFMT). Prise en charge en santé au travail des travailleurs intervenant en conditions hyperbares : Recommandations de bonne pratique Fiche de synthèse. Références En Santé Au Travail ; September 2016 ; N° 147 : 69-78

22. Société de Physiologie et de Médecine Subaquatiques et Hyperbares de langue française / Société Française de Médecine du Travail. Recommandations de bonne pratique : prise en charge en santé au travail des travailleurs intervenant en conditions hyperbares. Marseille: MEDSUBHYP and SFMT; Second edition 2018. 204 pages Available at URL https://www.medsubhyp.fr/images/consensus_bonnes_pratiques_reglementation/Sant-au-travail-des-travailleurs-hyperbares-2018-v2.pdf

23. Panchard MA, Bänziger O, Fuchs H, Haldi H, Oswald H. Recommendations for estimating diving ability in children .Pediatrica Vol. 17 No. 4 2006 [cited 10/3/ 2019] Available from URL http://www.swiss-paediatrics.org/sites/default/files/paediatrica/vol17/n4/pdf/10-14.pdf

24. Hugona M, Gemppa E, De Maistrea S, Lougea P, Pontierb J M, Pényc C et al. Aptitude médicale à la plongée autonome et au travail en milieu hyperbare dans les armées .Médecine et armées.2015 ; 43 (1): 13-8

25. D'Andréa C. Examen de non contre-indication à la plongée ARESUB meeting 8 August 2007 [on line : 22/06/2008] available at http://aresub.pagespersoorange.fr/medecinesubaquatique/medecineplongee/cipatho/examnonci.htm

26. Aqua med. Examination for fitness to dive. Aqua med Am Speicher XI 11 28217 Bremen Germany [Online]. May 2017 [cited 10/4/ 2019]; [2 screens] available from URL:https://www.aquamed.eu/fileadmin/documents/medicine/tauchtauglichkeit_fr.pdf

27. Wuillemin T, Bragança ADS, Lanier C, Berney JY, Ziltener JL. Medical certificates for stays in high mountains and scuba diving. Rev Med Suisse 2014; Vol 10.1772-8 available at URL https://www.revmed.ch/RMS/2014/RMS-N-443/Certificats-medicaux-pour-les-sejours-en-haute-montagne-et-la-plongee-sous-marine

28. - Health and Safety Executive HSE. The medical examination and assessment of commercial divers (MA1) [Online]. October 2015[citation date] : 27 pages available at http://www.hse.gov.uk/pubns

29. Coulange M, Barthélémy A. Certificat médical, contre-indications temporaires et définitives à la plongée. Science & Sports [Online]. 2012 April [cited 10/4/2019]; Volume 27, No. 2 [131-7] available from URL https://www.em-consulte.com/en/article/709133

30. Reynaud P, Certificats médicaux : la responsabilité médicale en matière de plongée sous-marine avec scaphandre Medical certificates: medical responsability in scuba diving Revue des Maladies Respiratoires. September 2001 ; Vol 18 N° 4 : p. 379 Available at URL https://www.em-consulte.com/rmr/article/143312

31. Professional Association of Diving Instructors PADI Medical fitness - candidate declaration 2pages Version 2.01 1/6 2014 Published on https://www.padi.com

32. Géraut C, Tripodi D, Géraut L. Risks of scuba diving and working in hyperbaric environments. Encycl Med Chir (Elsevier Masson, Paris) - Pathologie professionnelle et de l'environnement 2008:1-13 [Article 16-560-A-10].

33. Sames C, Gorman D, Mitchell S, Sandiford P. An evidence-based system for health surveillance of occupational diversions. Intern Med J. 2016 Oct;46(10):1146-52.

APPENDIX 1

Investigation into the medical certificate of fitness to dive

Data collection form

Confidential and anonymous form ***(Please circle the correct answers)***

1. **Age** (in years) ....
2. **Sex** □ H □ F

3. You are a diver

Professional Amateur Sportsman Other (specify)

3 bis In which region of Tunisia do you dive?

....

4 If professional, in which field do you work?

....

5. **How many years have you been diving?** ....

6. How often do you dive?

_____/ Week ____/ month ____/ year

7. **During your diving career, did you receive a medical certificate stating that you were fit (or not contraindicated) to dive?**

YES □ NO □

8. Your first medical certificate was issued in which year? ___________

9. **The certificate was issued by which category of doctor?**
   - General Practitioner
   - Sports doctor
   - Family doctor
   - Hyperbaric doctor
   - Specialist doctor ? ____________________

10. Have you subsequently obtained certificates of no contraindication to diving?

Yes □ No □

If yes, from which category of doctor did you obtain your certificate?

- General Practitioner
- Sports doctor
- Family doctor
- Hyperbaric doctor
- Specialist doctor ? ____________________

11. Generally, you will obtain your medical certificate of fitness to dive from a doctor :

- Du Privé, de libre pratique □
- A public health structure □

12. How often do you have your medical certificate for diving?

- Only once □
- Every 6 months □
- Every year □
- Every two years □
- Every five years □
- Other (please specify) ________________________________

13. During the medical consultation, did you have the following tests before receiving your medical certificate issued by the doctor?

▪ Blood tests	never	sometimes	Often	regularly
▪ Electrocardiogram ECG	never	sometimes	Often	regularly
▪ Chest X-ray	never	sometimes	Often	regularly
▪ ENT examination	never	sometimes	Often	regularly
▪ Respiratory function test	never	sometimes	Often	regularly
▪ Audiogram (hearing measurement)	never	sometimes	Often	regularly
▪ Impedance measurement (ears)	never	sometimes	Often	regularly
▪ Electroencephalogram EEG	never	sometimes	Often	regularly
▪ Radiography of the hips	never	sometimes	Often	regularly
▪ Shoulder X-ray	never	sometimes	Often	regularly
▪ Knee X-ray	never	sometimes	Often	regularly
▪ Compression test in hyperbaric chamber	never	sometimes	Often	regularly
▪ Exercise test never sometimes yes once often	never	sometimes	Often	regularly
▪ Other examination (please specify)				

14. Have you ever been involved in a diving accident?

Yes □ No Never □

If yes, describe what happened

....

....

15. Have you ever had one or more sessions in a hyperbaric chamber?

Yes □ No □

16. Comments

____

Thank you for your cooperation

APPENDIX 2

SAMPLE FTASS MEDICAL CERTIFICATE [4]

LEVEL 1 DIVING MEDICAL CERTIFICATE

I, the undersigned Doctor

....

Federal physician, Physician approved by the FAST CMP, certifies that I have examined the following on this day

Mr, Mrs:

....

And declares that he/she :

- didn't tell me about any pathological history
- is not medically contraindicated for scuba diving
- has no contraindications to the practice of underwater activities:
    - ....

The test must be repeated before:

....

Date: ....

Signature of legal representative Signature and stamp of doctor

Father, Mother, Guardian

NB: To prepare for the level 2 exam and beyond, the medical certificate must be drawn up by a Fédéral doctor or a doctor approved by FAST.

The trainee and the doctor certify that they are aware of the medical contraindications to diving listed overleaf.

CONTRAINDICATIONS for SCUBA DIVING

	Contre indications définitives	Contre indications temporaires
Cardiologie	Cardiopathie congénitale Insuffisance cardiaque symptomatique Cardiomyopathie obstructive Pathologie avec risque de syncope Tachycardie paroxystique BAV II ou complet non appareillés Maladie de Rendu-Osler Valvulopathies(*)	Hypertension artérielle non contrôlée Coronaropathies : à évaluer(*) Péricardite Traitement par anti-arythmique :à évaluer(*) Traitement par bêta-bloquants par voie générale ou locale: à évaluer (*) Shunt D G découvert après accident de décompression à symptomatologie cérébrale ou cochléo-vestibulaire(*)
Oto-rhino-laryngologie	Cophose unilatérale Évidement pétromastoïdien Ossiculoplastie Trachéostomie Laryngocèle Déficit audio. bilatéral à évaluer (*) Otospongiose opérée Fracture du rocher Destruction labyrinthique uni ou bilatérale Fistule peri-lymphatique Déficit vestibulaire non compensé	Chirurgie otologique Épisode infectieux Polypose nasosinusienne Difficultés tubo-tympaniques pouvant engendrer un vertige alterno-barique Crise vertigineuse ou au décours immédiat d'une crise Tout vertige non étiqueté Asymétrie vestibulaire sup. ou égale à 50%(6mois) Perforation tympanique(et aérateurs trans-tympaniques) Barotraumatismes de l'oreille interne ADD labyrinthique +shunt D-G :à évaluer(*)
Pneumologie	Insuffisance respiratoire Pneumopathie fibrosante Vascularite pulmonaire Asthme :à évaluer (*) Pneumothorax spontané ou maladie bulleuse, même opéré : à évaluer(*) Chirurgie pulmonaire	Pathologie infectieuse Pleurésie Traumatisme thoracique
Ophtalmologie	Pathologie vasculaire de la rétine, de la choroïde, ou de la papille,non stabilisées, susceptibles de saigner Kératocône au delà du stade 2 Prothèses oculaires ou implants creux Pour les N3, N4 , et encadrants : vision binoculaire avec correction<5/10 ou si un œil<1/10,l'autre <6/10	Affections aigues du globe ou de ses annexes jusqu'à guérison Photokératectomie réfractive et LASIK : 1 mois Phacoémulsification-trabéculectomie et chirurgie vitro-rétinienne : 2 mois Greffe de cornée : 8 mois Traitement par béta bloquants par voie locale : à évaluer(*)
Neurologie	Épilepsie Syndrome déficitaire sévère Pertes de connaissance itératives Effraction méningée neurochirurgicale, ORL ou traumatique Incapacité motrice cérébrale	Traumatisme crânien grave à évaluer
Psychiatrie	Affection psychiatrique sévère Éthylisme chronique	Traitement antidépresseur, anxiolytique, par neuroleptique ou hypnogène Alcoolisation aiguë
Hématologie	Thrombopénie périphérique, thrombopathies congénitales. Phlébites à répétition, troubles de la crase sanguine découverts lors du bilan d'une phlébite. Hémophiles : à évaluer (*)	Phlébite non explorée
Gynécologie		Grossesse
Métabolisme	Diabète traité par insuline : à évaluer (*) Diabète traité par antidiabétiques oraux (hormis biguanides) Troubles métaboliques ou endocriniens sévères	Tétanie / Spasmophilie
Dermatologie	Différentes affections peuvent entraîner des contre-indications temporaires ou définitives selon leur intensité ou leur retentissement pulmonaire, neurologique ou vasculaire	
Gastro-Entérologie	Manchon anti-reflux	Hernie hiatale ou reflux gastro-œsophagien à évaluer

NB:

- Any medication taken must be assessed
- All pathologies marked with an (*) must be assessed, and the medical certificate of no contraindication can only be issued by a federal doctor or a doctor approved by FAST.
- The resumption of diving after a diving accident or incident will require the advice of a Federal Doctor or one approved by FAST.

APPENDIX 3

Recommended examinations to determine initial or periodic suitability for hyperbaric exposure

Occupational health care for workers in hyperbaric conditions Recommendations for good practice

Société de médecine et de physiologie subaquatiques et hyperbares de langue française (MEDSUBHYP). French Society of Occupational Medicine (SFMT) [21].

	Systematic examinations			Examinations on indication
	Initial examination	Annual review	Five-year review	
General examination				
Self-questionnaire Thorough clinical examination BMI	x x x	x x x	x x x	
Pneumology				
Recording flow-volume curves	x	after 40 years	x	Chest CT, full EFR (non-mobilisable volumes, TLCO, bronchial reactivity 1, stress test)
ENT				
Otoscopy with Valsalva manoeuvre Pure tone audiometry	x x	x if exposed to noise	x x	Complementary vestibular investigations
Cardiology				
Thorough clinical examination with measurement of resting blood pressure Resting ECG Assessment of adaptability	x x questioning/ questionnaire	x after 40 questioning/ questionnaire	x x questioning/ questionnaire	MAPA Exercise test for subjects at risk (see p. 97) of the argument) Ultrasound Maximal exercise test with determination of ventilatory and

to exercise				metabolic thresholds
Musculoskeletal system				
Thorough clinical examination	x	x	x	MRI of joints
Ophthalmology				
Visual acuity with and without correction	x	x	x	Visual field Examination of transparent media
Neurology and psychiatry				
Appropriate questioning (history-taking) Thorough clinical examination	x x	x x	x x	EEG anxiety test Brain MRI and neuro-psychological assessment after the age of 40
Haematological disorders				
Clinical examination History taking CBC	x x x	x x	x x x	Search for thrombophilia
Dermatology				
Examin ation Clinical examina tion	x x	x x	x x	

1. *Metacholine challenge test or beta-2-mimetic aerosol reversibility test.*

Occupational health care for workers in hyperbaric conditions Recommendations for good practice

Société de médecine et de physiologie subaquatiques et hyperbares de langue française (MEDSUBHYP). French Society of Occupational Medicine (SFMT) [21].

BMI: body mass index; CT: computed tomography; EFR: functional respiratory examination; TLCO: capillary alveolar carbon monoxide transfer; ECG: electrocardiogram; MAPA: ambulatory blood pressure measurement; MRI: magnetic resonance imaging;

EEG: electroencephalogram; CBC: blood count; GFR (CKD-EPI): glomerular filtration rate (GFR) according to the CKD-EPI formula (Chronic kidney disease - Epidemiology collaboration).

	Systematic examinations			Examinations on indication
	Initial examination	Annual review	Five-year review	
Stomatology				
Appropriate history-taking Full endobuccal examination	x x x	x x x	x x x	Dental panoramic radiography
Gastroenterology				
Appropriate history-taking	x x	x x	x x	
Gynaecology - obstetrics				
Appropriate questioning	x	x	x	Pregnancy test Ultrasound if pregnancy in progress
Additional biological tests				
Fasting blood glucose Lipid profile Creatininaemia GFR assessment (CKD-EPI) Proteinuria test	x x x x x x	x	x x x x x x	Liver check-up Testing for psychotropic drugs in urine or blood

APPENDIX 4

Recommended examinations to investigate the long-term effects of exposure to hyperbaria (after the age of 40, on indication)

Occupational health care for workers in hyperbaric conditions Recommendations for good practice

Société de médecine et de physiologie subaquatiques et hyperbares de langue française (MEDSUBHYP). French Society of Occupational Medicine (SFMT) [21].

Target organs	Examinations	Anomalies sought	Comments
Lungs	Spirometry TLCO (on request)	Reduction in maximum flow rates, Tiffeneau coefficient, DEMM 25-50%, reduction in TLCO	Decrease in FEV1 and FVC after age 40
Brain	MRI (on request)	Hypersignals of the white matter, predominantly fronto-parietal	Number of hypersignals correlated with the presence of a large right-left shunt Complete with a neuro-psychological assessment
Device osteoarticular	MRI (on request)	Search for osteonecrosis, T1 hyposignal of the bone marrow	Preferential involvement of shoulders, hips and knees (MP no. 29 RG)
ENT	Pure tone audiometry	Sensorineural hearing loss	Not directly related to hyperbaria, but to the associated noise pollution
Eye	Fundus Visual field, Colour vision	Dysbaric retinopathy	Impaired colour vision, central visual field, degenerative lesions of the peripheral retina

TLCO: *alveolocapillary carbon monoxide transfer;* MMED: *median peak expiratory flow;* FVC: *forced vital capacity;*

FEV1: *forced expiratory volume in one second;* MRI: *magnetic resonance imaging;* OD: *occupational disease;* GP: *general health insurance scheme.*

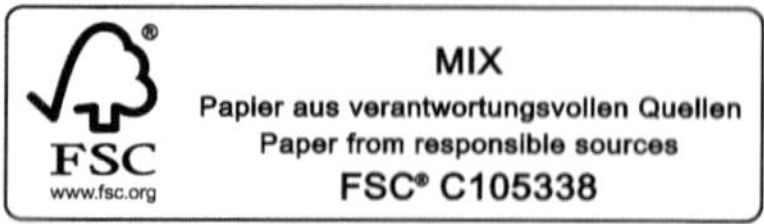

Printed by Books on Demand GmbH, Norderstedt / Germany